The Little Book of

Aphorisms & Quotations

for the Surgeon

Edited by
Moshe Schein

tfm Publishing Limited, Castle Hill Barns, Harley, Shrewsbury, SY5 6LX, UK
Tel: +44 (0)1952 510061; Fax: +44 (0)1952 510192
E-mail: info@tfmpublishing.com; Web site: www.tfmpublishing.com

Editing, design & typesetting: Nikki Bramhill BSc Hons Dip Law
Cover photo: © 2020 Evgeniy E. (Perya) Perelygin, MD

First edition:	© 2020
Hardback	ISBN: 978-1-910079-95-9
E-book editions:	2020
ePub	ISBN: 978-1-910079-96-6
Mobi	ISBN: 978-1-910079-97-3
Web pdf	ISBN: 978-1-910079-98-0

Printed by Gutenberg Press Ltd., Gudja Road, Tarxien, GXQ 2902, Malta
Tel: +356 2398 2201; Fax: +356 2398 2290
E-mail: info@gutenberg.com.mt; Web site: www.gutenberg.com.mt

Contents

Foreword   viii

Dedication   x

Abdominal surgery   1

Academia   7

Appendicitis   13

Assessment   16

Assistants, students & residents   19

Biliary   24

Cancer surgery   27

Colorectal surgery   31

Common sense   36

Complications   41

Critical care   55

Diagnosis   61

Dogma   66

Education   70

Errors   75

Ethics   80

General concepts	87
Hemorrhoids	103
Hernia	106
Innovations/gimmicks	109
Intestine	116
Judgment	120
Laparoscopy	132
Malpractice & law	144
Money matters	151
Obesity	156

Old age   160

Operating   166

Other disciplines   182

Pathology   187

Patients   191

Pilots vs. surgeons   199

Politics and admin   204

Practice   211

Research, writing, reading & publication 221

Surgeons   244

Thyroid & parathyroid 268

Vessels & amputations 271

Foreword

In the past, I have compiled two books of collected surgical aphorisms: the larger *Aphorisms & Quotations for the Surgeon*, with its 1500 quotations, and the slimmer *A Companion to Aphorisms & Quotations for the Surgeon*.

Since their publication, both books have become best-sellers. Surgeons use the books to 'decorate' their lectures or manuscripts with relevant smart or entertaining entries; some like to quote from the books during teaching rounds or conferences; many simply enjoy them for their collective and eternal surgical wisdom and wit.

Now, as I am drifting towards retirement, here is the last in the trilogy of this international bestselling series — *The Little Book of Aphorisms & Quotations for the Surgeon*. The quotes collected within this little book have been gathered since the publication of the last two books in the series.

As before, these aphorisms and quotations have been retrieved from multiple sources: journals, books, lectures and, more and more, gathered from surgical friends around the world.

The decision to include any entry is based on my personal taste. Some may question the wisdom or accuracy of individual entries; others may not 'get' the humor or may object to political incorrectness.

But I hope that most readers, especially younger surgeons, will discover that surgical truth is old, that what they think is a novel idea has been said before, and that what they observe around them — has been observed years ago. It may contribute to their humanity and humility, perhaps even add maturity to their surgical personality and practice. In addition, with a bit of luck, it may increase their sense of surgical humor — for how can one survive a lifelong surgical career without possessing some of it:

Common sense and a sense of humor are the same thing, moving at different speeds. A sense of humor is just common sense, dancing. Those who lack humor are without judgment and should be trusted with nothing.

Clive James (1939-2019)

Now let me conclude with a 'mother' of medical aphorisms:

From inability to let well alone, from too much zeal for the new and contempt for what is old, from putting knowledge before wisdom, science before art and cleverness before common sense, from treating patients as cases and from making the cure of the disease more grievous than the endurance of the same, good Lord deliver us.

Sir Robert Hutchison (1871-1960)

Good luck!

Moshe Schein MD FACS FCS (SA)
Ladysmith, Wisconsin

I wish to dedicate this book to

Professor David Dent

of Cape Town, South Africa:

a great surgeon, a wise man

and a master surgical aphorist!

ABDOMINAL SURGERY

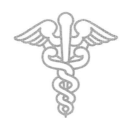

I cannot see what harm has been done if the appendix has been removed. The perfect man is the man without an appendix.

R. H. Harte (?1899)

If you don't eat, you don't shit.

If you don't shit — you die!

Barry (Baz) Alexander

Considering adhesionlysis: we were all schooled in not overdoing it with excessive enterolysis. In the laparoscopic era, it's often tempting to do adhesion release in the process of an otherwise routine lap cholecystectomy — possibly because it looks so dramatic with a pneumoperitoneum with adhesions on a string. It's like eating peanuts or snacking on potato chips (crisps for you Brits)... not knowing when to stop.

Angus Maciver

I divide interloop adhesions only if there is a discrepancy of size between loops.

Vinay Mehendale

Be careful with the knots, and do not damage the suture material with the instruments. The abdomen is like a big fish; a big fish can pull your knots and break your line – a distended abdomen can do the same.

Moshe Schein

ACADEMIA

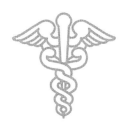

Scholarship is not what you happen to know about a subject; scholarship is what there is to know about that subject.

Harry Austryn Wolfson (1887-1974)

[About discussants at meetings]

While some are thoughtful, even dialectic, others are inappropriately sardonic, and others are without substance or relevance. Some of our colleagues rise for mere recognition of their presence at the meeting, while others go on record to have their abbreviated remarks listed (surprisingly enough) in their curriculum vita. A majority of discussants parade to the podium, often sitting in the rear of the hall, seldom using readily accessible floor microphones.

Claude H. Organ (1926-2005)

Let us remember that the responsibility of the discussant is not to 'stick it' to the presenter but to aid in the educational experience of the audience.

Jonathan van Heerden

Dr. Will Mayo many many years ago stated that every

lecture should fulfil 4 criteria:

1. Tell the audience what you are going to tell them;

2. Tell them;

3. Tell them what you have just told them;

4. Keep it short.

Jonathan van Heerden

I have evolved two inviolate rules for meetings:

1. Never go to a session if you

don't understand the title;

2. Avoid all short paper sessions

unless your resident is speaking.

Mark Cheetham

APPENDICITIS

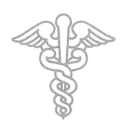

There are three types of patients with acute appendicitis: those who do well no matter what we do; those who don't do well no matter what we do; and those in whom our management actually makes a difference. As most fall into the first category... every surgeon believes that what he does is the right thing to do.

Magnus Bergenfeldt

More than 100 years after the first appendectomy the natural history of untreated acute appendicitis is unknown.

ASSESSMENT

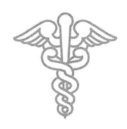

*'O*pen' referees' reports are not worth the paper they are written on. They usually convey the idea that the candidate is a blend of Michael de Bakey, Albert Schweitzer and Sister Theresa. Closed and 'confidential' ones are also rather fulsome; perhaps they fear the candidate may see them? On the other hand, well targeted phone calls yield amazing info, some good and some dirt.

David Dent

Oddly in the U.S. we seem to have an aversion to writing anything in anybody's evaluation that is bad; we would rather cloak it in 'nice wording' and hope that the person reading it gets the undertone. For example, a student who is a loudmouthed braggart who does not take criticism well would be evaluated as "independent" or "has strong opinions". Someone who is lazy as hell would be evaluated as "nice personality" or "laidback". The worst thing is if you are labeled as "a pleasure to work with" without any other specific positive comments. Program directors know this is bad news.

Karen Draper

ASSISTANTS, STUDENTS & RESIDENTS

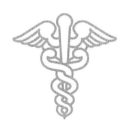

The best surgical assistant is mute, catatonic, and transparent.

Charles G. Rob (1913-2001)

I'm on a high-protein diet today.
I just chewed a resident's butt.

James H. Duke (1928-2015)

To medical students in the OR:

just allow a peek but not a poke!

Andy Gage

Hell has a special place for lousy assistants.

Dean Lutrin

BILIARY

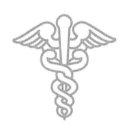

When I was a resident all GBs with stones were "chronic cholecystitis". In my early years all GBs without abnormal findings were "normal" (no surgeon ever liked this). In my mature years if I see two lymphocytes kissing it's "chronic cholecystitis"! I don't know any surgeons who take out normal GBs unless it was just in the way.

Miles J. Jones

Jaundice is 'medical' when you are too surgically focused, and 'surgical' when you are too medically focused.

B. Ramana

CANCER SURGERY

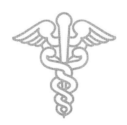

Telling a radical node resecting surgeon that his results are mere artefact, due to a powerful stage migration effect, is like telling a radical religious person that their views are flawed.

David Dent

Nor breast nor colon nor stomach.

Chasing lymph nodes in adenocarcinoma is

like obliterating the tire marks where the

car has been. It's the mets that kill;

no one has ever died of nodes.

David Dent

There is no evidence that lymph node removal alters prognosis at any site. The axillary debates in breast cancer are merely storms in an armpit.

David Dent

COLORECTAL SURGERY

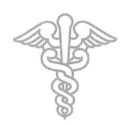

Certainly perianal Crohn's disease can look alarming; however, the temptation to treat alarming appearances with aggressive surgery must be resisted if the situation is not to be made worse by iatrogenic morbidity.

Allan A. Keighley

Fistula-in-ano surgery is challenging. Unlike most surgery where success rates are compared, fistula surgery is assessed by failure rates!

John Thanakumar

As I tell all my patients I know when the colonoscope is in the rectum and the ileum but ensuring any location anywhere else in the colon is a crapshoot. So even if you are God's gift to colonoscopy, mark the site of bleeding.

Jonathan Efron

It's funny that the patient poops and the surgeon is relieved.

Amjad Siraj Memon

COMMON SENSE

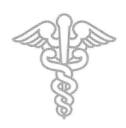

Common sense in not commonly practiced nowadays, particularly when it goes against the recommendation of 'experts'.

Samir Johna

Evidence is the base of medicine but common sense is the salt of it.

Slava Ryndine

No sensor should be allowed to completely replace common sense.

Kuldip Pandey

Common things are common except common sense.

Yasser Mohsen

COMPLICATIONS

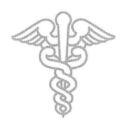

We hate complications even though they love us.

Hanafy Hanafy

Anastomotic leakage is a completely avoidable complication; providing you don't perform an anastomosis.

Brendan Moran

Those who opened the
retroperitoneum
on a renal fracture still
talk of this with
sobs in their voice.

B. Ramana

Surgeon: "It's amazing how the family members

of doctors always get complications."

Nurse: "But Doctor, all of your patients

get complications, you only remember

the family members of doctors."

Dean Lutrin

If it can get infected, it will.

Patrick A. Stone

If your stats are too good, just operate on a

health care professional's family member.

Patrick A. Stone

When things are going bad,

i.e. there's blood in the water,

don't wait to see the sharks to call for help.

Patrick A. Stone

*Ileus and wound infection
means a leak until proven otherwise.*

Dean Lutrin

The Shit Surgeon Syndrome (SSS): any postoperative

complication is blamed on a triad of:

a) Someone else — "the resident did the anastomosis";

b) The kit — "the new staple guns are shit";

c) The patient — "they were too fat".

We've all heard the same excuses a hundred times —

in my case frequently in my own head,

from the devil on my shoulder.

Simon Shaw

I used to get angry when we lost a patient until one day my chairman, Dr. Jack Bloch, gave me his take on it: "you cannot make chicken salad out of chicken shit."

Samir Johna

It doesn't matter what you put on a bedsore as long as it is not the patient.

10% of patients seem to get 90% of the complications.

Il medico pietoso fa la ferita infetta — the pitiful doctor makes the wound infected.

CRITICAL CARE

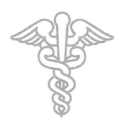

This is the reality of intensive care: at any point, we are as apt to harm as we are to heal.

Atul Gawande

An extra hour of shit in the abdomen – an extra day in the ICU.

John Edington

About CPR:

If you can't keep them alive

when they're alive,

you can't keep them alive

when they're dead.

Angus Maciver

The patient is in intensive care but still alive.

Javier Pérez de Cuéllar

The C *in the ATLS ABC*

is for CIRCULATION

– not for CHOPPER.

Moshe Schein

DIAGNOSIS

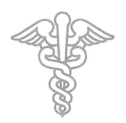

Beware of the surgeon with only one differential diagnosis.

John Santaniello

It sounds better in German:

"Wer viel misst, misst viel mist" –

people who test too much tend to get bullshit.

Lope Estévez-Schwarz

The certainty that scores give to clinicians who like to see themselves endowed with higher knowledge from hand-held devices is more than often frustrated by the stubbornness of individual patients who refuse to follow the way of the score.

Erik Schadde

We used to use the abbreviation exam NAD

(no abnormality detected)

but now I suspect it is exam NAD

(not actually done!).

John Leslie

DOGMA

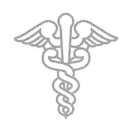

He believes in evidence-based surgery,
except when he doesn't.

B. Ramana

Blind adherence to old dogma is like adhesions following surgery. They cause obstruction, nausea, vomiting, pain, and constipation.

Francis Seow-Choen

How many unfounded dogmas – things which we are doing without 'evidence' – are now being studied over and over again – to prove that the unproven things are unproven.

Moshe Schein

EDUCATION

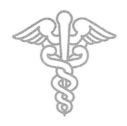

The great vice of medical education is its tendency to fix attention on the latest and the best only, to the neglect of what has been accomplished in the past. At times, the latest book on a subject is not the best… this comes chiefly for lack of knowledge of previous experience.

Leslie Cowlishaw (1877-1943)

I cannot, for the life of me, figure out why the hours of surgical education are getting easier while the surgical pathology we seek to eliminate is getting more difficult.

Leo Gordon

There is an analogy here to the

self-esteem movement in education.

Educators are afraid of hurting the student's self-esteem.

If this continues, students will feel better and

better about knowing less and less.

The result is a graduate who feels great

about knowing nothing.

Leo Gordon

During the first ten years you learn how to do the surgery; the next ten years you learn when to perform surgery, and in the last ten years you learn when to refrain from surgery.

Kuldip Pandey

ERRORS

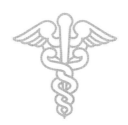

You must learn from the mistakes of others. You can't possibly live long enough to make them all yourself.

Sam Levenson (1911-1980)

I always prefer to be open and honest about my mistakes.

There is an art to doing this, as you know.

When one falls on the sword,

the sharks tend to swim away.

When one is defensive, it tends to chum the waters.

Bob Goldman

You are less likely to commit an error if you consider an atypical presentation of a common condition than a typical presentation of a rare condition.

Wojciech J. Górecki

To err is human – this adage always seems 'correct' if the error has been committed by yourself, or one of your buddies – the error appears much less 'human' if inflicted on you, or one of your dear ones.

Moshe Schein

ETHICS

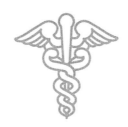

The prime goal is to alleviate suffering, and not to prolong life. And if your treatment does not alleviate suffering, but only prolongs life, that treatment should be stopped.

Christiaan Barnard (1922-2001)

I had bought two male chimps from a primate colony in Holland. They lived next to each other in separate cages for several months before I used one as a [heart] donor. When we put him to sleep in his cage in preparation for the operation, he chattered and cried incessantly. We attached no significance to this, but it must have made a great impression on his companion, for when we removed the body to the operating room, the other chimp wept bitterly and was inconsolable for days. The incident made a deep impression on me. I vowed never again to experiment with such sensitive creatures.

Christiaan Barnard (1922-2001)

It is infinitely better to transplant a heart than to bury it to be devoured by worms.

Christiaan Barnard (1922-2001)

Almost all medical professionals have seen what we call "futile care" being performed on people. That's when doctors bring the cutting edge of technology to bear on a grievously ill person near the end of life. The patient will get cut open, perforated with tubes, hooked up to machines, and assaulted with drugs. All of this occurs in the ICU at a cost of tens of thousands of dollars a day. What it buys is misery we would not inflict on a terrorist.

Ken Murray

*U*nder the cover of science, innovation, progress and surgical solutions to non-surgical issues, patients are still serving as mice in our experiments. Informed consent is a joke when we ourselves are so clueless.

Danny Rosin

In some ways the true face of any society

is reflected not by its army, movie industry,

internet connectivity, media, stock exchange,

car industry, number of senators

or congressmen — but how well it

looks after the sick and poor.

Moshe Schein

GENERAL CONCEPTS

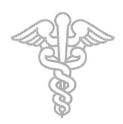

I would say that major surgery includes all work
requiring a general anesthetic; all operations which
involve openings into the great cavities of the body; all
operations in the course of which hazards of severe
hemorrhage are possible; all conditions in which the life of
the patient is at stake; all conditions which require for
their relief manipulations, for the proper performance of
which special anatomic knowledge and manipulative skill
are essential. …You will see that there is still left an
abundant field for the practitioner of minor surgery.

Lewis S. Pilcher (1845-1934)

The final success of an operation does not depend upon the suture material but upon the power of tissue to unite.

George Grey Turner (1877-1951)

Surgery has no parallel in human experience. The violent intrusion into the body of an accepting fellow-being for the ultimate benefit of the violated is a powerful experience. After continued repetition, some surgeons become muddled as to which party has the rights and which the privilege.

N. S. Mitchell

Patients never die of fluid overload on the medical service or dehydration on the surgical one.

Timothy C. Fabian

The 4 Rs on how to deal with surgical stress: Religion; Romance; Running; Red wine.

John Bruni

One of our great failings is to reduce management into binary possibilities. You do, or you don't; you give, or you don't give; it is black or it is white.
Nature, disease, patients and outcomes are, however, a spectrum of possibilities. So, too, should our management be, and that includes antibiotics for diverticular disease.

David Dent

As I tell the students, a lot of things about surgery really suck, but it is still the best job in medicine, and it has a history, amusing anecdotes, etc. Plus we get to work on the coolest thing on the planet, the human body, and most of the time if we don't violate some pretty simple basic rules, it heals just fine and patients are happy.

Albert I. Alexander

Surgical self-esteem is a fundamental knowledge of surgical pathology coupled with the skills to treat that pathology. Achieving that self-esteem takes time and effort. It does not conform to a clock or a schedule.

Leo Gordon

Two of the most powerful therapeutic agents in surgery are time, and natural history.

David Dent

We have all heard of "evidence-based medicine". But let's not ignore "enteric-based medicine" –
the thought 'in your gut' that this is doing some good.

Leo Gordon

The snowball effect of rescue procedures,

and the different attitudes of the different groups involved:

Rescue teams — get 'em to hospital alive;

ER — get 'em out of here alive;

OR — get 'em to the ICU alive;

ICU — we must keep 'em alive whatever.

But who sees the overall picture?

Barry (Baz) Alexander

As you know, holding fire is much more difficult than shooting. This is true for the police force, the Marines, the IDF and surgeons.

Moshe Schein

Avoid the fog of transfer.

An asymptomatic patient is likely to become symptomatic after the operation.

Magnitude of bleeding:
see, hear, or feel…

HEMORRHOIDS

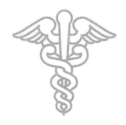

The similarity between smartphones and piles: ultimately every asshole gets one.

Vinay Mehendale

Prolapsed hemorrhoids:

if you let it subside spontaneously

the patient will have pain for 7 days,

but if you operate the pain will last a week.

Simon Shaw

Hernia

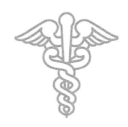

The humble umbilical hernia remains a simple yet complex issue.

Lawrence T. Kim

Laparoscopic umbilical hernia repair is like going to the center of the earth to plant a seed near the surface.

Rolando Ramos

INNOVATIONS/GIMMICKS

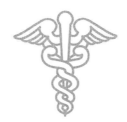

Every year sees methods of treatment tried

over again which were tried and found

wanting many years before, and fresh discoveries

vaunted which are only rediscoveries.

This waste of effort and time arises from ignorance

of what has been accomplished before.

Leslie Cowlishaw (1877-1943)

I don't believe medical discoveries are doing much to advance human life. As fast as we create ways to extend it we are inventing ways to shorten it.

Christiaan Barnard (1922-2001)

NOTES

(natural orifice transluminal endoscopic surgery) is NUTS.

SILS

(single-incision laparoscopic surgery) is SILLY.

Mark Cheetham

Soon there will be a specialist for the right nostril and another specialist for the left one. However, when a casualty is admitted with a wound of both nostrils, until the two specialists arrive, there will be no more nose left.

Moshe Hashmonai

This procedure is very good.
Yes, it has a long learning curve.
You have to f*** up a large number of
unsuspecting patients before you
can master it.

Kuldip Pandey

There are many factors determining if a change in practice will 'catch' on. Saving money, doing less, and thinking more are not among the immediate suspects.

Danny Rosin

INTESTINE

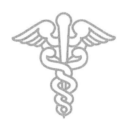

In my experience, the diagnosis of gastroenteritis in the emergency ward is often incorrect as to raise a serious question whenever the emergency physician comes to this conclusion.

Zachary Cope (1881-1974)

I would rather leave a piece of mesh on the bowel than a piece of bowel on the mesh.

Moshe Schein

Beware of the diagnosis of gastroenteritis in the elderly.

JUDGMENT

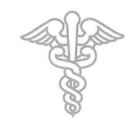

The surgeon who strives for perfection

needs some basis for patient selection.

He would like to be sure

there's a good chance for cure

before he starts the resection.

Elwood G. Jensen

Surgeons frequently have tunnel vision which only sees the nail, which they are tempted to smite with a hammer; they do not see the whole structure behind it, or ask why the nail is protruding.

David Dent

Evidence-based clinical decision-making may require input from a multidisciplinary group of experts, as opposed to a 'consensus of one'.

Laurent G. Glance

It is judgment not genital insufficiency driving a surgeon to pack his patient's abdomen.

David J. Richardson

Some correct decisions cannot be judged by retrospective knowledge.

Danny Rosin

The first thing to go when you are tired is your judgment.

Dean Lutrin

It's better to be an optimist who is sometimes wrong than a pessimist who is always right.

John Leslie

He used to tell his patients while

taking consent for any operation

"Sir or Madam, I am a pessimistic realist."

Not the worst thing to be for a surgeon.

Mathias Kalkum

Indications can be stretched like chewing gum or the brain of surgeons. Unfortunately arteries are not as pliable.

Moshe Schein

Clinical experience has been defined as making the same mistake with increasing confidence for an impressive number of years in contrast to evidence-based medicine which involves perpetuating other people's mistakes instead of your own.

One of the rarest things that we do is think. I don't know why people don't do it more often. It doesn't cost anything. Think about that.

LAPAROSCOPY

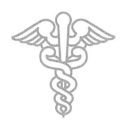

Laparoscopy shares many similarities with the emperor's cloth. If you do not join in the choir of praises, you are either stupid or unfit for the job. But someone needs to tell the truth.

Roland Andersson

Laparoscopic surgery is the one case where a resident can destroy the remainder of a patient's life, and your mental health and well-being with one squeeze of the clip applier or one cut of the shears.

Jeffrey Young

Even in teaching, laparoscopy takes longer than open surgery.

John Santaniello

A rule of thumb is that the tumour should be removed by laparotomy and not laparoscopy if it is bigger than the head of the surgeon in question.

David Dent

If you can't do it with the laparoscope alone,

you shouldn't do it with the robot.

If you can do it with the laparoscope,

you don't need the robot.

Mark Pleatman

Laparoscopic cholecystectomy: a nickel and dime operation with a million dollar complication.

Nathaniel Soper

The most important aim of cholecystectomy

is not to injure the CBD;

the second most important aim

is to relieve any sepsis;

the third — if it can be done safely — is to

remove the gallbladder.

Kristoffer Lassen

Laparoscopy is a path, not a goal.

The goal is a safe outcome.

Vinay Mehendale

I know lots of anaesthetists who rely upon anecdote to judge us surgeons. Almost to a man (or a woman) they regard laparoscopic surgery as a means by which straightforward operations that used to be done quickly now take hours and inevitably involve vast quantities of disposable kit.

John MacFie

I never saw a patient dying because he was converted to open; I saw them dying because they were not converted.

Moshe Schein

Laparoscopic cholecystectomy should take as long as it takes to do it safely; and if it takes too long it only means that the surgeon should have attempted subtotal cholecystectomy or 'converted' to open earlier.

Moshe Schein

Malpractice & Law

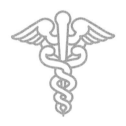

Informed consent is not the piece of paper, it is the process of understanding, and the agreement.

David Dent

Shit happens, but the patient needs

to be given some reasonable money;

lawyers must not get ANY money;

the surgeon must not be made out to be a criminal.

Court time and resources need to be used properly.

Anil Thakur

Shit does happen but it comes usually from arseholes.

Barry (Baz) Alexander

I am amazed, in every trial I've had, how a jury can see through a difficult situation and find for the doctor if two things are proven to them: first, you know what you're doing, which is easy to prove, and second, that you care. If we are able to prove that to the jury, they will excuse the most unbelievable things.

Curtis Diedrich

The increasingly politically correct medical system wishes us to "hear no evil, see no evil, do no evil". The results: evil is being committed, people see it but pretend they do not; they speak about it — but behind the back.

Moshe Schein

The "standard of care" is a good place to hide if you don't have a better idea and the talent to execute it.

MONEY MATTERS

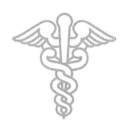

The principal object of the patient is to get cured; the principal object of the surgeon is to get paid.

Henri de Mondeville (1260?-1320)

There are only four forms of incentive that I now, in my 27th year as a surgical chair, recognize: cash, money, cash money, and everything that can be converted into cash money.

Josef E. Fischer

Patients are viewed as biological cash-producing units, with a cynical reimbursement system that makes it all the more lucrative. The system works like this everywhere.

Jon Lloyd

One of the things about the U.S. health care system is that it defies the laws of economics, and of gravity. Once the price is high, it just stays there.

Naoki Ikegami

OBESITY

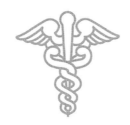

If the poor overweight jogger only knew how far he had to run to work off the calories in a crust of bread he might find it better in terms of pound per mile to go to a massage parlor.

Christiaan Barnard (1922-2001)

*F*or the vast majority of patients today, there is

no operation that will control weight to a 'normal'

level without introducing risks and side effects that

over a lifetime may raise questions about its use

for surgical treatment of obesity.

Edward Mason

There are no difficult operations,
only fat people.

Stephen Clifforth

Old Age

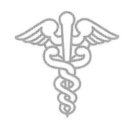

When a surgeon is old enough to have experience that's all he's got going for himself.

Matt Paneth (1921-2011)

It's just that as an old general surgeon, I usually reserve optimism until the day after discharge, or often until the first post-op visit. Until then I plan for the next worst potential problem.

Jerry Kaplan

They say that a surgeon's 'expiry date' is tattooed on the back of his neck where he can't see it, but everyone else can.

David Dent

There is nothing like a major operation to make someone show their real age.

Jeffrey Matthews

The 'generational gap' between today's

young and old surgeons:

*the young need to **see** everything;*

*the old have to **feel** everything.*

Moshe Schein

OPERATING

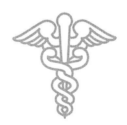

*T*here is no value to an operation
that only one surgeon can do.

Berkeley George Andrew Moynihan (1865-1936)

Classification of an operation according to Moosa:

Type I — a difficult operation made to appear easy;

Type II — a difficult operation made to look even more difficult by the operator;

Type III — an easy operation made to look difficult.

May you always have Type Is.

Abdool R. Moossa (1939-2013)

Meticulous surgical technique:
a touch of a lady; allergic to blood.

Jonathan van Heerden

A small scar doesn't matter in the coffin.

Ari Leppäniemi

The key is to make an incision.

If it is the wrong incision,

then make another incision.

Matthew Reeds

SLICE surgery:

Single Large(r) Incision

Cost-Effective surgery.

David Wattchow

I once asked my boss why he tied his knots seven times: "Last time I did six, it didn't hold."

Bernard Cristalli

There is slow and there is slow.

It can result from slow, continuous, confident

and accurate movements, or from unnecessary

repetitive, inaccurate and ineffective movements.

I accept the first option as fully legitimate;

the second is not to be praised.

Danny Rosin

If you haven't seen it done before, there is a reason why.

Patrick A. Stone

If you don't like how it looks like today

— you sure won't tomorrow.

Patrick A. Stone

The first scary experience you will encounter:

when you look across the table and

realize that you are the most

experienced surgeon in the room.

Patrick A. Stone

You want a fast trauma surgeon and a slow cancer surgeon.

Dean Lutrin

In Sweden we say:

"Går det lätt så är det rätt,

är det rätt så går det lätt."

If it is easy, it's the right thing to do,

if it's the right thing to do, it will be easy.

Roland Andersson

"Find safety in the heart of danger"
— unveil the hidden traps so as better
to avoid them or control them.

Kristoffer Lassen

*There are two rules to safe surgery
– see what you are doing and
leave a dry field.*

OTHER DISCIPLINES

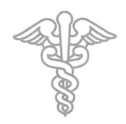

When the internist wants an operation –

think twice.

And make sure you do the correct one,

not what he suggests.

And if he doesn't –

then there may be a real indication.

Danny Rosin

An orthopedic surgeon and an internist

trying to stop the elevator:

the internist puts his hand in the door;

the orthopedic surgeon puts in his head.

Hand surgeon:
one who wants to put his
hand on all cases.

The rectal tone of the anesthesiologist varies with the patient's O_2 saturation.

PATHOLOGY

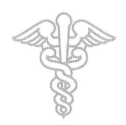

The only thing more complex than human pathology is the system we have designed to identify and to treat human pathology.

Leo A. Gordon

$$A \; x \; P = c.$$

The Law of Anatomy and Pathology

states that the product of anatomy and

pathology equals a constant: the more

pathology you have, the less anatomy you get.

Amram Ayalon

The more complex the pathology – the simpler the surgical solution should be.

Moshe Schein

PATIENTS

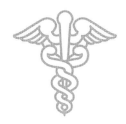

When a patient writes a letter of praise it should not be read, but that when a letter of the opposite type is received, in which our demerits are carefully depicted, we should go over it with great care, because we would probably learn something.

Charles Mayo (1865-1939)

You can listen your way into your patients' lives better than you can talk your way into that relationship.

Antonia Novello

It is often the difficult patient who survives,

when the submissive and suffering good

patient dies of natural causes or medical errors,

because these difficult patients tend

to have a fighting spirit.

Bernie Siegel

There is nothing biologically different about a pope or a president, and there is no need to alter one's thinking in caring for them.

Jay A. Block

I find that an increasing percentage of my practice is dedicated to convincing patients they don't need the operation they were referred for, and relieving their anxiety after being exposed to horror stories of what can happen.

Danny Rosin

The operation is not over until the patient is home eating his favorite meal.

Dean Lutrin

*To reassure the patient
you must be sure.*

PILOTS VS. SURGEONS

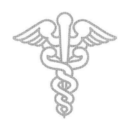

*P*ilots may have more incentive than surgeons

to be perfect, right or wrong.

When they botch a landing, it's usually their last.

Fortunately, modern day aircraft are a lot

more predictable and reliable than any of our patients.

Any pilots will tell you that.

Tim Eldridge

Pilots don't fill out a form documenting that they put a landing gear down. This is another fundamental difference in the two professions. We (surgeons) obsess about documentation; aviation worries about getting the wheels down.

Richard C. Karl

I do know that it is harder to control bleeding from the back side of the portal vein than it is to land a 737 with an engine on fire.

Richard C. Karl

*If you deviate from a rule
(e.g. 'standard of care'),
it must be a flawless performance
(e.g. if you fly under a bridge,
don't hit the bridge).*

POLITICS AND ADMIN

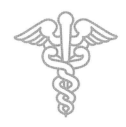

Clichés, stock phrases, adherence to conventional, standardized codes of expression and conduct have the socially recognised function of protecting us against reality; that is, against the claim on our thinking attention which all events and facts make by virtue of their existence.

Hannah Arendt (1906-1975)

Administrators become Executive Directors, etc., until they finally arrive as "President and C.E.O.". Joe boys and girl fridays get sequentially elevated to "Vice President"...in charge of such bizarre portfolios as "patient experience", "strategic corporate planning", "interprofessional relations"...wtf is next? Vice President of Laundry, Vice President of Food Services, Vice President of Parking... They breed like maggots feeding off a decaying corpse.

Angus Maciver

The furies that populate committees, requiring more and more documentation, that reduce the time for one on one connections… we become detached from those who become 'problems' and 'cases', rather than unique fellow humans.

Barry (Baz) Alexander

Advice from an old fart: play the facts not the person.

Matt Oliver

Ideal hospital for the administrators:

no doctors, no patients, lots of money.

Ideal hospital for the doctors:

many patients, lots of money, no

administrators.

Bernard Cristalli

Try to attend important meetings; if not at the table you will be on the menu.

PRACTICE

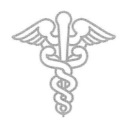

The concept that one citizen will lay himself horizontal and permit another to plunge a knife into him, take blood, give blood, rearrange internal structures at will, determine ultimate function, indeed, sometimes life itself — that responsibility is awesome both in true and in the currently debased meaning of that word.

Alexander J. Walt (1923-1996)

*U*nfortunately, the practice of surgery today is as much a business as it is a science and art.

Thomas R. Russell (1940-2014)

Doctors live in a sea of ignorance surrounding small islands of knowledge that sustain us until another island appears.

Daniel C. Wilkerson, Jr. (1922-2017)

When I use the words "bad situation" I am implying an unfavorable outcome, unless you recognize that for hundreds of years physicians considered an early death in futile situations as the most favorable outcome. When God puts Her/His hands on, take yours OFF.

Kenneth Mattox

Y ou can often get away with a less safe process, but that doesn't mean it is safe; it just means that you got away with it.

Jeffrey Young

Politically correct, PC, is an artificial behavioural code that is transient; good manners and sensitivity are a basic behavioural code that should be permanent.

David Dent

One could compare the practice of surgery to

having unprotected sex with a beautiful whore:

you have fun for an hour or so...

then you worry, worry, worry —

and occasionally you suffer.

Moshe Schein

Less is more unless it isn't.

Excellent results don't just happen —
they are earned.

RESEARCH, WRITING, READING & PUBLICATION

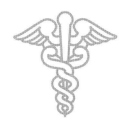

Billings' rules for scientific authors:

1. Have something to say;

2. Say it;

3. Stop as soon as you have said it;

4. Give the paper a proper title.

John Shaw Billings (1838-1913)

*There is a dead medical literature
and there is a live one.
The dead is not all ancient,
the live is not all modern.*

Oliver Wendell Holmes (1841-1935)

I would advise the young surgeon to write papers and in writing to bear in mind what the old minister said: "few souls are saved after the first 25 minutes of the sermon." Write the paper not to show how learned you are, or to show the high type man who may be in the audience, that you are in his class. Rather, try to tell those in your audience who perhaps may not know as much about the subject as you, something that may interest and help them. Do not try too many points.

William Mayo (1861-1939)

To the young surgeon I would say, do not read all surgery and technique, for technique is constantly changing. Along with surgical literature, read medical articles in high-class medical journals. Do not skim, but here and there select certain articles and read them with care.

William Mayo (1861-1939)

Statistical numbers are like prisoners of war – torture them enough and they will admit to anything.

Basil A. Pruitt (1930-2019)

A rule of thumb: a retrospective study proves nothing but generates a hypothesis to be proven.

Lew Flint

As far as the surgical literature goes, use the "Texas mockingbird approach": eat everything in sight and vomit what you can't use.

Lew Flint

A difference, to be a difference,
must make a difference.

Lew Flint

If you can't see a clinically significant difference, it probably isn't there regardless of what the statistics say.

Lew Flint

My scepticism is, however, greatest with observational studies from single centres, with famous individual reporters.

David Dent

Statistics is like a bikini: what it shows you is very interesting but what it doesn't is far more interesting!

Samir Johna

To my mind, the trialists (similar to the big pharmas in medicine and device manufacturers in surgery) have hijacked the EBM train and as some would say changed "evidence-based medicine" to "evidence-biased medicine".

Saba Balasubramanian

In surgery, you don't get to revise. In writing, you are revising all the time and you are constantly striving to do something new. If I started following a formula with my writing, everyone will know it and it will fail. In surgery, you are trying to do, as much as possible, the same things over and over again, and to perfect what you do, I like having both.

Atul Gawande

Researchers headed into their studies wanting certain results — and lo and behold, they are getting them. We think of the scientific process as being objective, rigorous, and even ruthless in separating what is true from what we merely wish to be true. But in fact it's easy to manipulate results, even unintentionally or unconsciously… at every step of the process there is room to distort results, a way to make a stronger claim or to select what is going to be concluded. …there is an intellectual conflict of interest that pressures researchers to find whatever it is that is most likely to get them funded.

John Ioannidis

As a general rule, results of observational studies should be taken with a grain of salt. Otherwise, one might conclude that gray hair causes heart attacks.

Edward H. Livingston

Your essays should be like women's skirts — long enough to cover the subject but short enough to be interesting.

Ms. Jane Ray [Cited by Leo Gordon]

Editorials are not meant to tell readers what to think but to tell them what to think about.

Richard Smith

It may be that their data pass the t-test, but they don't pass the so-what test.

Erik Schadde

The absence of evidence isn't the evidence of absence.

Henry Black

*Only bad writers think that
their work is really good.
This applies to surgeons as well.*

Moshe Schein

Definition of a double-blind randomized trial:
two surgeons reading an ECG.

Gratis asseritur, gratis negatur. That which is asserted without evidence may be denied without explanation.

Surgeons

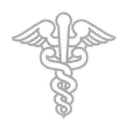

A very ordinary surgeon, by means of selection of cases, aseptic care, and the kindness of nature, may have a low death rate, and yet benefit his patients but little.

Charles Mayo (1865-1939)

Chloroform has done a lot of mischief.

It's enabled every fool to be a surgeon.

George Bernard Shaw (1856-1950)

From my surgical teacher, the late Prof. Sir John Bruce, at the University of Edinburgh: "There is no minor surgery, just minor surgeons."

Joe Lemer

Even a drunken pig will occasionally find a truffle.
This applies to surgeons as well.

Rob Lane

The surgeon's ego does not always recognise when it has been abusive, exploitive or patronizing. It does not adapt easy to the new ethos of the 90s which heralds teamwork, participative decision-making and decentralised responsibility.

N. S. Mitchell

I have many colleagues, all of varying levels of knowledge and skill. But the ones I trust most are the ones that worry. You can see the concern, sometimes even anguish on their faces. Then... there are the sociopaths...

Tom Gilas

Not analysed, seldom discussed, and rarely published,

is the reality that there are good cutting surgeons

and bad cutting surgeons. Yes, broadly — two kinds.

Outside of these normal parameters, there are

also wizard cutting surgeons and surgical butchers.

This was, and is, and ever will be.

David Dent

On the surgical ego:
It is nice to be important, it is much more important to be nice.

Jonathan van Heerden

About surgeons:

Few professionals are more willing

to discuss, or have more fun discussing

patients without expecting financial

remuneration for this discourse.

Jonathan van Heerden

Do you know the surgical definition of 'colleague'? A person that has exactly the same profession as me but is a little less good at it.

Danny Rosin

Definition of a modern surgeon: one whose ignorant opinion is evidence-based.

B. Ramana

As an historic legacy, surgeons feel obliged to add a few zeroes religiously against the number of operations they have done. For example, you will rarely find an Indian surgeon who has done less than 15,000 LCs.

B. Ramana

There are two types of female surgeons:

there are surgeons who shouldn't be female

and females who shouldn't be surgeons.

Mark Pleatman

After 33 years in the surgery I observe a lot of very happy surgeons, most of them stopped reading medical journals after graduation; they have no complications, they know everything and they are informed only by company representatives handing out glossy brochures.

Marian Littke

The four phases of evolution of a surgeon:

1. A surgeon feels insecure and this is justified (beginning of training);

2. A surgeon feels confident but this is not justified

(dangerous for the patients...);

3. A surgeon feels confident and it is justified

(after years of training, alas some never reach this stage);

4. And the final stage as the surgeon grows old

(he feels insecure but it is not justified).

Alexander Schoucair

Surgeons are influenced by their most recent pleasant or unpleasant experience.

Kenneth Mattox

A rich man's faults are covered with money, but a surgeon's faults are covered with earth.

Abraham Verghese

Nothing is as holy to the surgeon as is his own skin.

Klaus Henner Laue

Big surgeons are those who are not too big to deal with the small things.

Moshe Schein

A successful surgeon should be a man who, when asked to name the three best surgeons in the world, would have difficulty deciding on the other two.

Denton Cooley (1920-2016)

I was thinking that surgeons had to be the happiest people on earth. To cut people up and get paid for it — that's happiness, I told myself.

Norman Mailer (1923-2007)

As a surgeon you have to have a controlled arrogance. If it's uncontrolled, you kill people, but you have to be pretty arrogant to saw through a person's chest, take out their heart and believe you can fix it. Then, when you succeed and the patient survives, you pray, because it's only by the grace of God that you get there.

Mehmet Öz

At a given instant everything the surgeon knows suddenly becomes important to the solution of the problem. You can't do it an hour later, or tomorrow. Nor can you go to the library and look it up.

John W. Kirklin (1917-2004)

THYROID & PARATHYROID

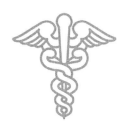

If the superior gland is missing, look inferior to the inferior for the superior; and if the inferior is missing, look superior to the superior for the inferior gland.

Jonathan van Heerden

Has the patient renal stones.

Painful, brittle, broken bones.

Complaints of thirst and constipation.

Next to peptic ulceration.

And you doubt his mental state.

Determine calcium and phosphate.

Sure the underlying the mechanism.

Might be hyperparathyroidism.

Hajo A. Bruining

Vessels & Amputations

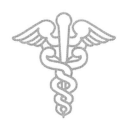

Make claudicators beg for intervention.

Patrick A. Stone

Amputation survival is equivalent to metastatic cancer.

Patrick A. Stone